How To Master Digital Bird Photography

A Comprehensive Guide

JOHNSON WU

ISBN 978-1-998455-95-9 (Paperback)

ISBN 978-1-998455-96-6 (eBook)

Printed and bound in USA

Published by Loons Press

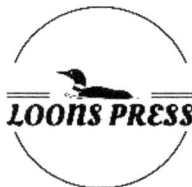

LOONS PRESS

Table Of Contents

How To Master Digital Bird Photography

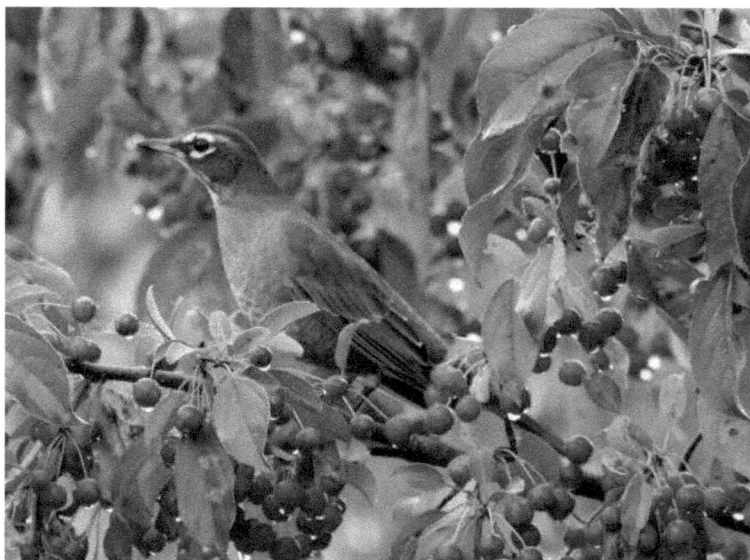

Chapter 1

Introduction to Bird Photography

The Allure of Bird Photography

The allure of bird photography lies in its unique blend of challenge and reward. Capturing the essence of a bird in its natural habitat requires not only technical skills but also a deep understanding of avian behavior.

Photographers often find themselves immersed in the beauty of nature, waiting patiently for that perfect moment when a bird takes flight, lands gracefully, or engages in a captivating display of courtship. This pursuit can be both exhilarating and meditative, as it encourages a connection with the environment and fosters a greater appreciation for wildlife.

One of the most compelling aspects of bird photography is the diversity of species and their behaviors. With over 10,000 bird species worldwide, each presents its own set of challenges and opportunities. From the vibrant plumage of tropical birds to the stark elegance of raptors, every photograph tells a story. Understanding the habitats and behaviors of different species can significantly enhance the quality of the photographs. This knowledge allows photographers to anticipate actions, such as feeding, nesting, or mating, which can lead to striking images that capture the essence of avian life.

Bird photography also serves as a gateway to conservation awareness. As photographers document the beauty and intricacies of various species, they often become advocates for their protection. The images produced can highlight the fragility of ecosystems and the impact of human activity on wildlife.

By sharing their work, photographers can inspire others to appreciate and protect avian species, fostering a sense of responsibility towards conservation efforts. This aspect of bird photography creates a meaningful connection between the photographer and the broader environmental community.

The technical demands of bird photography further enhance its allure. Mastering the intricacies of camera settings, lenses, and lighting conditions can be both challenging and rewarding. Photographers must develop a keen eye for composition while also being prepared to adapt quickly to changing conditions.

The necessity for specialized equipment, such as telephoto lenses and sturdy tripods, adds a layer of excitement to the pursuit. Each outing presents new opportunities to refine skills, experiment with different techniques, and ultimately create stunning images.

Lastly, the social aspect of bird photography enriches the experience. Many photographers find camaraderie in shared interests, joining clubs, attending workshops, and participating in online forums. This community fosters an environment of learning, support, and inspiration. Sharing tips, techniques, and experiences not only enhances individual skills but also cultivates friendships built around a mutual passion for capturing the beauty of birds. The allure of bird photography, therefore, extends beyond the act of taking pictures; it encompasses a holistic experience that connects individuals to nature, each other, and the world of conservation.

Understanding Bird Behavior

Understanding bird behavior is fundamental to mastering digital bird photography. Birds exhibit a range of behaviors that can provide photographers with insights into the best moments to capture stunning images.

By observing their habits, you can anticipate actions such as feeding, mating, and nesting, enabling you to position yourself for optimal shots. Each species has unique behavioral traits, and familiarity with these can significantly enhance your photography experience.

One of the key aspects of bird behavior is understanding their feeding patterns. Many birds have specific times of day when they are most active in search of food. Early morning and late afternoon are often peak feeding times. Observing these patterns not only helps in planning your photography outings but also increases your chances of capturing dynamic images.

For example, you might witness a hummingbird hovering over a flower or a raptor hunting from above. Knowing where and when to find these behaviors can lead to more successful and rewarding photography sessions.

Social interactions among birds also provide excellent opportunities for captivating photographs. Birds engage in various social behaviors, from mating displays to territorial disputes. Observing these interactions can reveal the best moments to click the shutter.

For instance, courtship rituals often involve elaborate displays that can be visually stunning. By understanding the social dynamics of the birds you are photographing, you can anticipate these moments and be ready to capture them in action.

Seasonal changes significantly affect bird behavior, influencing migratory patterns and breeding cycles. During migration, birds may congregate in large numbers, creating opportunities for breathtaking shots of flocks in flight. In contrast, breeding seasons often bring about increased territorial displays and nesting behaviors.

By timing your photography sessions according to these seasonal changes, you can take advantage of unique opportunities that arise, such as capturing the first moments of hatchlings leaving the nest.

Lastly, patience and persistence are essential elements in understanding bird behavior. Birds can be unpredictable, and it may take time to observe and learn their routines. Spending extended periods in the field allows you to become familiar with their movements and habits.

This investment in time often pays off with spectacular photographs that reflect not just the beauty of the birds but also the intricacies of their behavior. By committing to this process, you will not only improve your skills as a photographer but also deepen your appreciation for the avian world.

Essential Equipment for Beginners

When embarking on the journey of digital bird photography, understanding the essential equipment is crucial for beginners. The right gear not only enhances your ability to capture stunning images but also makes the process more enjoyable and efficient. At the core of your setup should be a good camera. A DSLR or mirrorless camera with interchangeable lenses offers the versatility needed for various shooting conditions. Look for models with fast autofocus systems and high burst rates, as these features are vital for capturing birds in motion.

Equally important is the lens. For bird photography, a telephoto lens is essential, allowing you to get close-up shots without disturbing the birds. A lens with a focal length of at least 300mm is often recommended for capturing clear images of birds from a distance.

Image stabilization can also be beneficial, especially when shooting handheld, to reduce the effects of camera shake. As you gain experience, consider investing in a longer lens or a teleconverter to further extend your reach.

In addition to the camera and lens, a sturdy tripod or monopod can significantly improve your photography. These tools provide stability, which is particularly important when using longer lenses that can be challenging to hold steady.

A tripod is ideal for static shots, while a monopod offers more mobility when tracking birds in flight. Look for options that are lightweight and easy to transport, as you may find yourself hiking or moving through various environments to find the perfect shot.

A quality camera bag is another essential item for beginners. It should be spacious enough to accommodate your camera, lenses, and other accessories while providing adequate protection against the elements. Water-resistant features are particularly useful, as bird photography often takes place in unpredictable weather conditions.

Additionally, consider including a rain cover for your gear, ensuring that you can continue shooting even during light rain or drizzle.

Finally, don't overlook the importance of memory cards and extra batteries. Bird photography can be unpredictable, with fleeting moments that require quick reflexes. Carrying multiple high-capacity memory cards ensures you won't miss a shot due to a lack of storage. Likewise, having extra batteries on hand allows you to shoot for extended periods without worrying about running out of power.

By assembling this essential equipment, beginners can lay a strong foundation for their bird photography endeavors, setting the stage for a rewarding and creative experience.

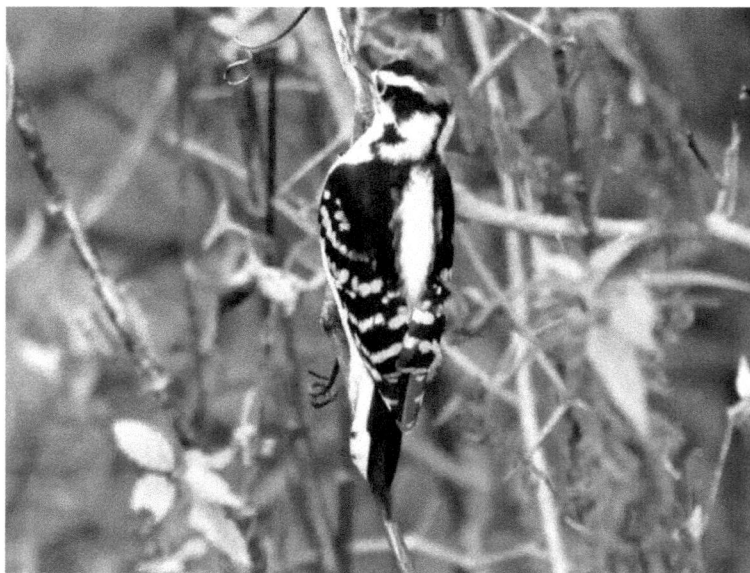

Chapter 2

Choosing the Right Camera

Types of Cameras for Bird Photography

When it comes to bird photography, selecting the right type of camera is crucial for capturing stunning images. There are several types of cameras available, each with its own set of features and advantages. Understanding these options can help you make an informed decision that aligns with your specific needs and photography style.

Common types of cameras for bird photography include DSLRs, mirrorless cameras, compact cameras, and superzoom cameras.

Digital Single-Lens Reflex (DSLR) cameras are a popular choice among bird photographers due to their versatility and performance. These cameras typically feature larger sensors, which allow for better image quality, especially in low-light conditions. The ability to change lenses enables photographers to use long telephoto lenses, which are essential for capturing distant birds.

Additionally, DSLRs offer fast autofocus systems and high frame rates, making it easier to track moving subjects. However, they can be bulky and heavy, which may be a consideration for those who prefer a more portable option.

Mirrorless cameras have gained significant popularity in recent years and are becoming a favorite among bird photographers. These cameras offer many advantages similar to DSLRs, such as interchangeable lenses and high-quality images.

The key benefit of mirrorless technology is the absence of a mirror mechanism, resulting in a more compact and lightweight design. This can be particularly advantageous for bird photographers who spend long hours in the field. Mirrorless cameras also feature electronic viewfinders, allowing for real-time exposure adjustments, which can be beneficial when photographing birds in varying lighting conditions.

Compact cameras, also known as point-and-shoot cameras, provide a more accessible option for those who may not want to invest in more complex systems. While they generally have smaller sensors, advancements in technology have resulted in compact models that produce impressive image quality. Some compact cameras come with powerful zoom lenses, making them versatile for capturing birds at various distances.

However, the limitations in manual control and slower autofocus may make it challenging to capture fast-moving subjects. Compact cameras are ideal for casual bird watchers who want to document their sightings without the burden of heavy gear.

Superzoom cameras offer a unique blend of features suitable for bird photography, combining the convenience of a compact camera with an extended zoom range. These cameras have built-in lenses that can cover a wide focal length, allowing photographers to capture close-up shots of birds without needing to change lenses.

The convenience of a superzoom camera makes it an attractive option for those who want to travel light while still having the capability to photograph birds at a distance. However, the image quality may not match that of DSLRs or mirrorless cameras, especially at higher zoom levels.

Therefore, it's essential for photographers to consider their priorities when selecting a camera for bird photography.

Key Camera Features to Consider

When choosing a camera for bird photography, several key features significantly affect the quality of your images and your overall shooting experience. The first feature to consider is the sensor size. A larger sensor typically captures more light and detail, which is crucial when photographing fast-moving birds in varying lighting conditions.

Full-frame sensors are ideal but may be costly; however, crop sensors can also deliver excellent results, particularly when paired with the right lens. Understanding the differences between sensor sizes will help you make an informed decision based on your budget and shooting style.

Another critical aspect is the autofocus system. Birds are often unpredictable and quick, so a camera with a fast and accurate autofocus system is essential. Look for features like multiple autofocus points and advanced tracking capabilities. Cameras with phase-detection autofocus will generally perform better in dynamic shooting situations. Additionally, consider the camera's ability to focus in low light, as early mornings or late evenings can provide some of the best birding opportunities.

Continuous shooting speed is another factor that directly impacts your ability to capture the perfect moment. A camera that can shoot at a high frames-per-second (FPS) rate allows you to take multiple shots in quick succession, increasing your chances of getting that elusive shot of a bird in flight or during a dramatic action sequence. Aim for a camera that can shoot at least 5 FPS, but higher is always better if you want to freeze fast action reliably.

Image stabilization is also an important feature to keep in mind, especially when photographing birds at long distances. Even the slightest camera shake can lead to blurred images. Many cameras come with built-in stabilization systems, while others rely on stabilized lenses. If you plan to shoot handheld, particularly with telephoto lenses, investing in a camera or lens with effective stabilization can greatly improve your results, allowing for sharper images even in challenging conditions.

Finally, consider the lens compatibility and available options for the camera you choose. Bird photography often requires long focal lengths, so ensure that your camera can accommodate a range of telephoto lenses that suit your shooting needs.

Some manufacturers offer specialized lenses designed specifically for wildlife photography, which can provide the sharpness and reach you need.

Researching the available lenses and their performance will enable you to create a versatile kit that can adapt to different birding scenarios.

Lens Selection for Bird Photography

When it comes to bird photography, lens selection is one of the most critical decisions a photographer can make. The type of lens chosen can significantly impact the quality of images captured, as well as the ease with which a photographer can work in the field.

Bird photography often requires specific focal lengths and features that enhance the ability to capture fast-moving subjects in various environments. Understanding the different types of lenses available and their respective advantages is essential for anyone looking to excel in this niche.

Telephoto lenses are the go-to choice for bird photographers, as they allow for close-up shots from a distance without disturbing the subjects. A focal length of 300mm or longer is generally recommended, as this range provides the necessary reach to photograph birds in their natural habitats.

Lenses in the 400mm to 600mm range offer even greater capabilities, allowing photographers to capture stunning details of birds while maintaining a safe distance. Additionally, prime lenses often provide superior image quality and wider apertures, making them ideal for low-light conditions, which are common in early morning or late afternoon birdwatching sessions.

Zoom lenses also have their place in bird photography, especially for those who prefer flexibility in framing their shots.

A good quality zoom lens with a range of 100-400mm or even 150-600mm can be advantageous, allowing photographers to quickly adjust their composition without changing lenses. This versatility can be particularly useful in dynamic environments where birds are constantly moving.

However, it is important to consider the trade-offs; zoom lenses may not always match the sharpness and low-light performance of prime lenses, but they can provide the convenience of capturing various subjects in different scenarios.

In addition to focal length, other factors such as image stabilization and autofocus capabilities play a significant role in lens selection. Image stabilization helps to reduce the effects of camera shake, which is especially important when using longer focal lengths.

Fast and accurate autofocus systems are crucial for capturing birds in flight or during sudden movements. When selecting a lens, photographers should look for models with advanced autofocus features and reliable stabilization to enhance their shooting experience and improve their chances of getting the perfect shot.

Finally, considering the weight and size of the lens is essential for bird photographers who spend extended periods outdoors. A heavy lens can lead to fatigue, making it challenging to maintain focus and composure while shooting.

Photographers may want to explore options that strike a balance between portability and performance. Additionally, using tripod collars and monopods can help stabilize heavier lenses while allowing for easier mobility.

Ultimately, careful lens selection tailored to individual shooting styles and preferences will greatly enhance the ability to capture breathtaking images of birds in their natural environments.

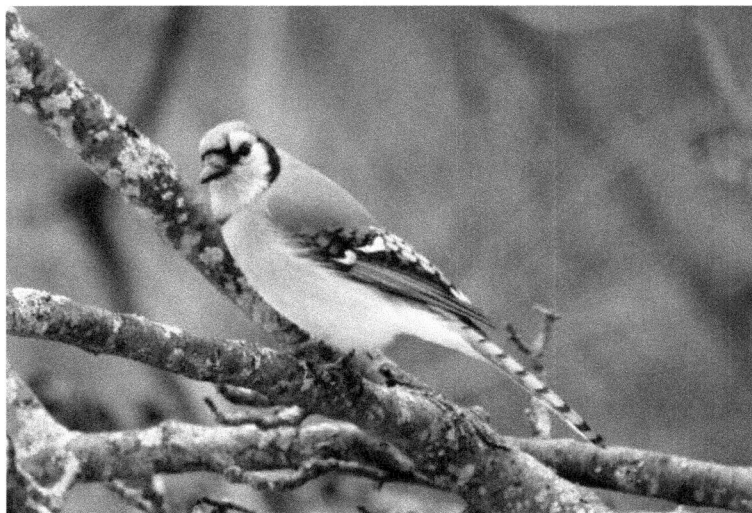

Chapter 3

Understanding Exposure

The Exposure Triangle: ISO, Shutter Speed, Aperture

The exposure triangle is a fundamental concept that every photographer must understand to capture stunning images. It consists of three key elements: ISO, shutter speed, and aperture. Each component plays a crucial role in determining the exposure of an image—the amount of light that reaches the camera sensor—and affects the overall quality of the photograph.

Understanding how these elements interact allows you to control the exposure creatively and achieve the desired results in your bird photography.

ISO refers to the sensitivity of your camera's sensor to light. A low ISO setting, such as 100 or 200, is ideal for bright conditions, producing images with minimal noise and high detail. However, during low-light situations, such as early morning or late evening when birds are most active, a higher ISO may be necessary to maintain a fast shutter speed and avoid motion blur.

While increasing the ISO can help in these scenarios, it's essential to be aware of the noise that can accompany higher settings. Striking a balance between ISO and light conditions is crucial for achieving clear, vibrant images of birds.

Shutter speed determines how long the camera's shutter remains open to capture light. Faster shutter speeds, like 1/1000 of a second, are essential for freezing the motion of birds in flight or capturing quick movements, such as a bird taking off or landing.

Conversely, slower shutter speeds can create interesting effects, such as motion blur, but they also increase the risk of camera shake, which can lead to blurry images. For bird photography, it is often recommended to use a shutter speed that is at least equal to the focal length of your lens to compensate for any potential blurriness caused by hand-holding the camera.

Aperture, represented by f-stops, controls the size of the lens opening that allows light to enter the camera. A wider aperture (lower f-stop number) not only lets in more light, which is beneficial in low-light situations but also creates a shallow depth of field. This is particularly useful in bird photography, as it helps isolate the subject from the background, making the bird stand out in the frame. A smaller aperture (higher f-stop number) increases the depth of field, allowing more of the scene to be in focus, which can be beneficial in certain compositions, especially when photographing birds in their natural habitats.

Mastering the exposure triangle is essential for any aspiring bird photographer. By understanding how ISO, shutter speed, and aperture work together, you can make informed decisions when adjusting your camera settings. This knowledge allows you to adapt to various lighting conditions and creatively capture the beauty of birds in flight or perched in their environments. Practicing with these three elements will help you develop your unique style and improve your overall skills, ultimately leading to captivating images that showcase the grace and elegance of birds.

Managing Exposure in Varying Light Conditions

Managing exposure in varying light conditions is crucial for capturing stunning bird photographs. Birds often inhabit diverse environments, from sun-drenched open fields to shadowy forested areas, each presenting unique challenges for photographers.

Understanding how to adjust your camera settings and make use of light effectively can significantly enhance the quality of your images, ensuring that the birds are well-exposed against their backgrounds.

In bright sunlight, the main challenge is often overexposure. The bright highlights can lead to loss of detail in the feathers and other features. To counteract this, photographers should consider using a faster shutter speed to freeze motion while also adjusting the aperture to limit the amount of light reaching the sensor. Using exposure compensation can help in reducing brightness, allowing for greater detail retention.

Additionally, shooting in RAW format provides the flexibility to recover highlights during post-processing, which can be particularly useful when working in harsh lighting conditions.

Conversely, in low-light situations such as early mornings or cloudy days, capturing details can be a challenge. Increasing the camera's ISO setting can help achieve a proper exposure, but it is essential to balance this with noise management. A higher ISO can introduce graininess to the image, so finding the optimal setting is key. Using a wider aperture can also aid in allowing more light into the camera, thereby improving exposure without sacrificing shutter speed too drastically.

A tripod or a stable surface can be beneficial in these situations to prevent camera shake, especially when using slower shutter speeds.

Backlighting is another common challenge when photographing birds. This occurs when the light source is behind the subject, often resulting in silhouettes. To manage backlighting effectively, photographers might need to adjust their position or use fill flash to illuminate the bird.

Additionally, employing exposure compensation can help in capturing the details of the subject rather than allowing the background to dominate the image. Experimenting with different angles and compositions can also yield interesting results, turning a potential problem into an opportunity for creativity.

In mixed lighting conditions, where both shadows and bright highlights exist, it becomes essential to analyze the scene carefully. Metering can be done through spot metering to ensure that the exposure is based on the bird itself rather than the surrounding environment. Utilizing bracketing techniques can also be advantageous, allowing photographers to take multiple exposures of the same scene to ensure that they capture the best possible image. Understanding how to manipulate light and exposure settings will enable photographers to adapt to varying conditions, leading to more dynamic and compelling bird photographs.

Exposure Compensation Techniques

Exposure compensation techniques are essential tools for photographers looking to enhance their images, particularly in challenging lighting conditions. In bird photography, where subjects can often be cloaked in shadow or overexposed by bright backgrounds, understanding how to manipulate exposure compensation can make a significant difference. This technique allows photographers to adjust the exposure level determined by the camera's metering system, ensuring that the details in both highlights and shadows are preserved.

One of the primary methods of exposure compensation is adjusting the exposure value (EV) settings on your camera. By increasing the exposure compensation, you can brighten your image, which is particularly useful when photographing birds against bright skies or reflective surfaces.

Conversely, reducing the exposure compensation can help prevent overexposure when the bird is set against a darker background. Mastering this adjustment gives photographers greater creative control, allowing them to achieve the desired mood and detail in their shots.

Another aspect to consider is the importance of understanding the metering modes available on your camera. Evaluative or matrix metering provides a comprehensive assessment of the entire scene, while center-weighted and spot metering focus on specific areas.

When photographing birds, using spot metering can be advantageous, especially when the subject is small compared to the background. This technique ensures that the exposure is based solely on the bird, leading to more accurate results and preventing the background from influencing the overall exposure.

In addition to camera settings, using exposure bracketing can be an effective way to capture the best possible image. This technique involves taking multiple shots at different exposure levels, allowing the photographer to select the optimal image later. Exposure bracketing is particularly beneficial in high-contrast situations, such as when birds are perched in dappled sunlight.

By capturing a range of exposures, photographers can ensure that they have options to work with, increasing their chances of achieving a perfectly balanced image.

Lastly, it is essential to practice and develop an intuitive sense for when to apply exposure compensation. Familiarity with the behavior of light in different environments can significantly enhance a photographer's ability to predict how adjustments will affect their images.

Regularly experimenting in various lighting conditions helps photographers refine their skills, allowing them to make quick and effective exposure adjustments in the field, ultimately leading to stunning bird photographs.

How To Master Digital Bird Photography

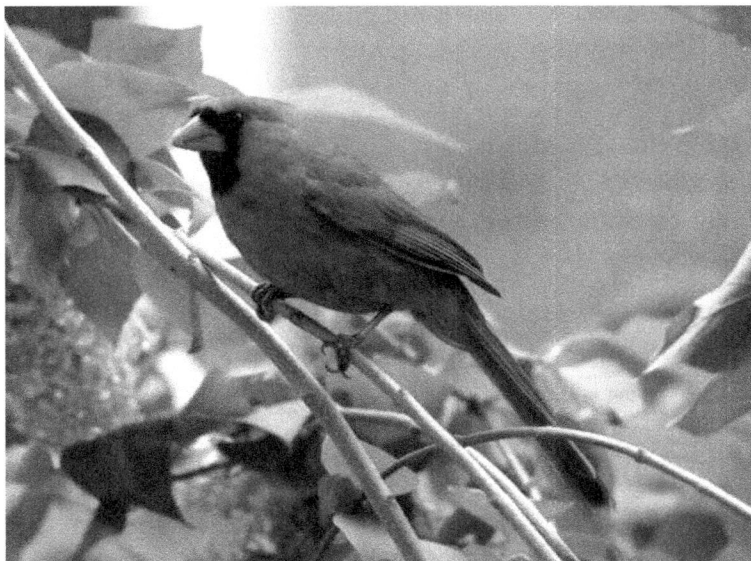

Chapter 4

Mastering Focus Techniques

Autofocus vs. Manual Focus

Autofocus and manual focus are two primary focusing methods that photographers can utilize, each with its distinct advantages and challenges. Autofocus systems have become increasingly sophisticated in modern cameras, employing various technologies such as phase detection and contrast detection to achieve quick and accurate focus. This feature is particularly beneficial in bird photography, where subjects can move unpredictably and often require rapid adjustments. Many photographers appreciate the convenience of autofocus, especially when trying to capture fleeting moments, such as a bird in flight or a sudden change in behavior.

While autofocus can be highly effective, it is not without its limitations. Autofocus systems can struggle in low-light conditions or when faced with complex backgrounds that confuse the camera's detection algorithms. In situations where a bird blends into its environment, such as a camouflaged species, relying solely on autofocus may lead to missed opportunities.

Additionally, autofocus may sometimes lock onto the wrong subject, particularly if multiple birds are in close proximity. Understanding these limitations is crucial for photographers aiming to capture sharp, well-focused images.

On the other hand, manual focus offers a level of control that can be advantageous in certain scenarios. Skilled photographers can precisely adjust focus to highlight specific details, such as a bird's eye or feathers, enhancing the overall composition.

Manual focus is particularly useful in macro photography or when shooting through obstacles like branches or foliage, where autofocus might struggle. By using manual focus, photographers can ensure that their attention is directed exactly where they want it, allowing for creative expression that may be lost when relying on automatic systems.

Choosing between autofocus and manual focus often depends on the photographer's style and the specific circumstances of the shoot. Many experienced bird photographers advocate for a hybrid approach, using autofocus for fast-moving subjects while switching to manual focus when precision is paramount. This combination allows photographers to adapt to different situations, ensuring they are prepared for both spontaneous moments and meticulously planned shots. Understanding when to employ each method is key to mastering bird photography.

Ultimately, mastering the balance between autofocus and manual focus can significantly enhance a photographer's ability to capture stunning images of birds. By familiarizing themselves with both techniques, photographers can develop a more versatile skill set, enabling them to respond effectively to the dynamic nature of their subjects.

As with any aspect of photography, practice and experimentation are essential. With time, photographers will learn to recognize the strengths of each focusing method and apply them appropriately, resulting in more successful and captivating bird photography.

Focus Modes and Their Applications

Focus modes are essential tools that photographers can leverage to capture stunning images of birds in their natural habitats.

Understanding the different focus modes available on your camera can significantly impact the quality of your photographs. The primary focus modes include single autofocus (AF-S), continuous autofocus (AF-C), and manual focus. Each mode offers distinct advantages and is suited for different scenarios encountered in bird photography.

Single autofocus (AF-S) is ideal for capturing still subjects or when the bird is perched. In this mode, the camera locks the focus when the shutter button is pressed halfway, allowing for precise focus on the subject.

This is particularly useful when photographing birds that are stationary, such as a robin on a branch or a blue jay at a feeder. AF-S provides a sharp focus on the subject while giving the photographer the ability to compose the shot without worrying about the focus shifting unexpectedly.

Continuous autofocus (AF-C), on the other hand, is designed for moving subjects, making it a crucial mode for bird photographers. When using AF-C, the camera continuously adjusts focus as the bird moves, ensuring that the subject remains sharp even in flight. This mode is particularly beneficial when photographing fast-moving birds, such as hawks in flight or small songbirds darting through the trees.

By keeping the focus locked on the subject, photographers can capture the dynamic and often unpredictable movements of birds.

Manual focus is another option that photographers may consider, especially in challenging situations where autofocus may struggle. Scenarios such as low light conditions, dense foliage, or when capturing birds that are camouflaged in their surroundings can benefit from manual focus.

This mode allows photographers to take complete control of the focus, enabling them to fine-tune their settings for optimal clarity. While it requires a steady hand and a keen eye, manual focus can result in striking images that showcase the intricate details of a bird's plumage or the subtle play of light in its environment.

In addition to understanding these focus modes, photographers should also consider their application in conjunction with other camera settings. Shutter speed, aperture, and ISO all play a crucial role in achieving the desired outcome. For example, using a fast shutter speed in combination with AF-C can help freeze the action of a bird in flight, while a wider aperture can create a beautiful bokeh effect, isolating the bird from its background. By mastering focus modes and their applications, photographers can elevate their bird photography, capturing moments that resonate with both beauty and technical precision.

Achieving Sharp Images of Moving Birds

Achieving sharp images of moving birds is a challenge that many photographers face, but with the right techniques and equipment, it is entirely possible. The first step to capturing sharp images is understanding your camera's autofocus system. Most modern cameras come equipped with advanced autofocus features, including tracking modes that can follow moving subjects.

Familiarize yourself with these settings to ensure that your camera can lock onto a bird in flight, adjusting focus as it moves. Utilizing continuous autofocus (AF-C for Nikon or AI Servo for Canon) is essential when photographing birds in motion, as it allows the camera to continuously adjust focus as the subject moves within the frame.

Another critical aspect of achieving sharp images is selecting the appropriate shutter speed. Birds can move at astonishing speeds, and a slow shutter speed can result in motion blur. A good rule of thumb is to use a shutter speed that is at least equal to the focal length of your lens. For instance, if you are using a 300mm lens, aim for a shutter speed of 1/300 seconds or faster.

In situations where the bird is particularly fast, you may need to increase the shutter speed even further. Keep in mind that higher shutter speeds require more light, so you may need to adjust your aperture or ISO settings accordingly.

Stabilization is another key factor in capturing sharp images of moving birds. If your lens or camera body has built-in image stabilization, make sure it is activated, as this can help reduce camera shake when shooting handheld.

Additionally, using a tripod or monopod can provide extra stability, especially when photographing birds at a distance. However, if you are in a situation where mobility is crucial, such as following a bird in flight, a tripod may be cumbersome. In these cases, consider using a gimbal head that allows for smooth panning while maintaining stability.

Composition plays a vital role in achieving sharp images as well. Anticipating the bird's movements and positioning yourself accordingly can lead to more dynamic shots. Use the rule of thirds to create a balanced composition while allowing space for the bird to move within the frame.

When photographing birds in flight, try to capture them against a contrasting background, such as a clear blue sky or a lush green field. This not only helps the bird stand out but also emphasizes its movement, creating a more engaging image.

Finally, post-processing can enhance the sharpness of your images after the shot is taken. Utilizing software like Adobe Lightroom or Photoshop can help you refine the details and clarity of your photographs. Pay attention to the sharpening tools, but be cautious not to overdo it, as this can introduce noise and artifacts.

Additionally, carefully cropping your images can help eliminate distractions while drawing focus to the bird, further enhancing the overall sharpness and impact of your photograph. By mastering these techniques, you will be well on your way to capturing stunning, sharp images of moving birds in their natural habitat.

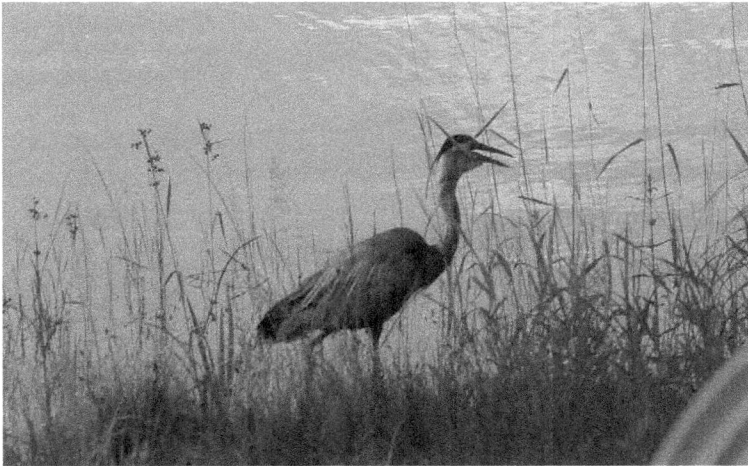

Chapter 5

Composition in Bird Photography

The Rule of Thirds and Beyond

The Rule of Thirds is a foundational principle in photography that enhances composition by guiding the placement of subjects within the frame. By dividing the image into nine equal parts with two horizontal and two vertical lines, photographers can position key elements along these lines or at their intersections. This technique helps create balance and draws the viewer's eye to the subject, making it particularly effective in bird photography, where dynamic movement and natural environments play a crucial role. Applying this rule can elevate your images, ensuring that your feathered subjects are not only prominent but also harmoniously integrated into their surroundings.

While the Rule of Thirds is a valuable starting point, it is essential to explore additional compositional techniques to enhance your bird photography further. Leading lines, for example, can guide viewers' eyes toward the subject, creating a sense of depth and movement. In the context of bird photography, elements such as branches, water lines, or paths can serve as natural leading lines that draw attention to the bird's position.

By actively looking for these lines in your composition, you can create a more engaging and visually appealing image that captures the essence of your subject and its environment.

Another compositional method to consider is the use of negative space. This technique involves leaving empty areas around your subject, which can create a sense of isolation or emphasize the bird's beauty.

In many cases, a bird in flight against an expansive sky or a solitary bird perched on a branch amidst a blurred background can evoke strong emotions and convey a sense of freedom. Utilizing negative space effectively can add drama and context to your photographs, allowing viewers to appreciate the subject while contemplating its surroundings.

Experimenting with different perspectives is also crucial in mastering bird photography. Instead of always shooting from eye level, try different angles and heights to create unique compositions. Low angles can make birds appear more majestic, while high angles can provide a broader view of the landscape. Additionally, varying your distance from the subject can yield different results; shooting close can capture intricate details, while a wider shot can place the bird in context with its habitat. Embracing various perspectives can lead to unexpected and compelling images that stand out in your portfolio.

Finally, as you become more comfortable with traditional compositional rules, consider breaking them intentionally to create bold, striking images. While guidelines like the Rule of Thirds serve as helpful tools, pushing beyond these conventions can lead to creative breakthroughs. Experiment with centering your subject, using symmetry, or incorporating unconventional framing techniques. Trust your instincts and artistic vision; sometimes, the most captivating bird photographs emerge when you step outside the box and embrace spontaneity in your approach.

Framing and Perspective Techniques

Framing and perspective techniques are essential components of capturing stunning bird photographs that stand out. Understanding how to frame a shot can transform an ordinary image into an extraordinary one.

When composing a photograph, consider the rule of thirds, which suggests dividing the frame into nine equal parts using two horizontal and two vertical lines. Positioning the subject along these lines or at their intersections can create a more engaging composition. Furthermore, incorporating natural elements like branches, leaves, or flowers can add depth and context, enhancing the viewer's connection to the scene.

Perspective greatly influences the viewer's experience of a photograph. Changing your position relative to the bird can yield vastly different results. For instance, shooting from a lower angle can create a dramatic effect, making the bird appear more imposing against the sky. Conversely, shooting from above can provide a unique view of the bird's behavior and surroundings. Experimenting with various heights and distances allows photographers to find the most compelling perspective, highlighting the bird's characteristics and its environment.

In addition to angle, focal length plays a critical role in framing and perspective. Telephoto lenses can isolate a subject by blurring the background, drawing attention to the bird itself. This technique is particularly useful for capturing details like feathers and eye color, which can be lost in wider shots.

However, using a wide-angle lens can also be effective, especially when aiming to capture the bird in its habitat. This approach provides context and tells a story about the environment the bird inhabits, making the photograph more engaging.

Lighting is another crucial factor that affects framing and perspective. The golden hours of early morning and late afternoon offer soft, diffused light that can enhance colors and textures in bird photography. Positioning yourself to take advantage of this natural light can significantly improve the quality of your images.

Additionally, backlighting can create a stunning silhouette effect, which can be particularly striking with certain bird species. Understanding how light interacts with your subject allows for creative framing opportunities that can elevate your photographs.

Finally, post-processing techniques can further refine framing and perspective in bird photography. Cropping an image can help eliminate distractions and focus the viewer's attention on the bird. Adjusting the perspective through software can correct any distortions caused by the lens and enhance the overall composition. While the goal should always be to capture the best possible image in-camera, digital editing provides an opportunity to fine-tune your work, ensuring that your photographs not only meet but exceed your artistic vision. Mastering these framing and perspective techniques can significantly enhance your bird photography, leading to images that resonate with viewers and convey the beauty of avian life.

Using Negative Space Effectively

Negative space is a crucial concept in photography that can dramatically enhance the visual impact of your bird images. In the context of digital bird photography, negative space refers to the areas surrounding your subject, which can help to emphasize the bird itself while creating a more balanced composition. By effectively utilizing negative space, photographers can draw the viewer's attention to the main subject and evoke a sense of tranquility and harmony within the frame.

When composing a shot, consider the placement of your bird within the frame. Positioning the subject off-center can create a greater sense of movement and direction, allowing the negative space to breathe and become an integral part of the composition.

This technique is particularly effective when photographing birds in flight or perched in a natural setting. The empty space surrounding the subject can suggest the bird's journey or its natural habitat, adding depth and context to your image.

Another aspect of using negative space is the choice of background. A simple, uncluttered background can enhance the effect of negative space, making the bird stand out more prominently. Look for backgrounds that contrast with the bird's colors or textures, ensuring that the subject remains the focal point.

This approach also aids in minimizing distractions that could detract from the overall impact of the photograph. A well-chosen background can transform an ordinary shot into an extraordinary one by emphasizing the beauty of the bird.

Lighting plays a significant role in how negative space is perceived in your photography. Soft, diffused light can enhance the mood and atmosphere of your images, allowing the negative space to take on a more significant presence.

Early morning or late afternoon light often provides a warm glow that can beautifully frame your subject and its surroundings. Experimenting with different times of day can help you discover how varying light conditions affect the relationship between your bird and the negative space.

Lastly, it is essential to practice and refine your understanding of negative space through regular experimentation. Review your images critically to assess how effectively you have used negative space in each shot. Look for opportunities to create images where the negative space adds meaning, context, and emotion to your work.

By continually challenging yourself to incorporate negative space into your compositions, you will develop a unique style that enhances your bird photography and resonates with your audience.

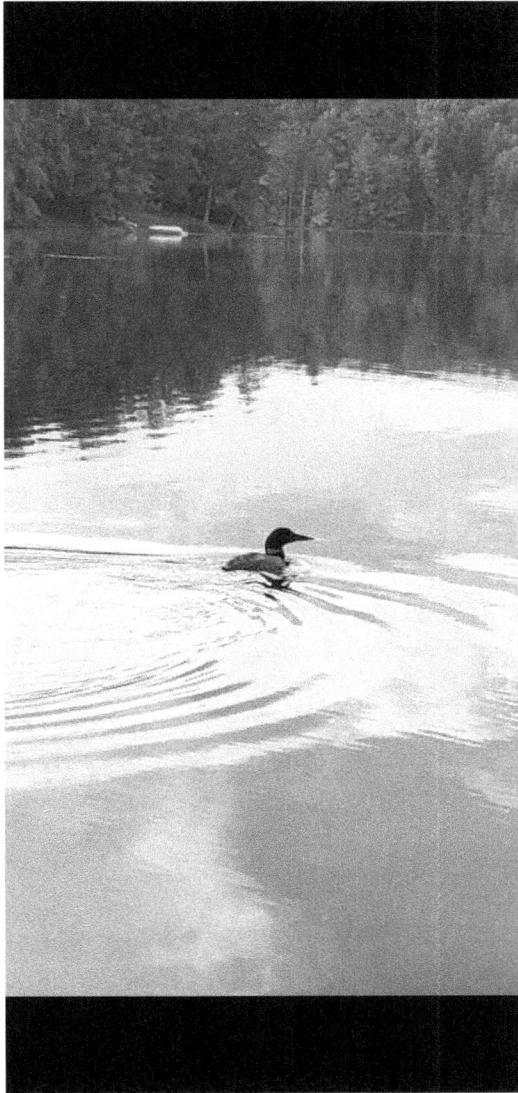

Chapter 6

Utilizing Natural Light

Best Times of Day for Bird Photography

The best times of day for bird photography are often dictated by the behavior of the birds themselves and the quality of natural light available for capturing images. Early morning and late afternoon are generally considered the prime times for bird photography.

During these hours, birds are most active, foraging for food, engaging in social behaviors, and preparing for nesting. The soft, golden light during sunrise and sunset not only enhances the colors in the feathers of the birds but also reduces harsh shadows, allowing for more flattering portraits.

Morning hours, particularly the first two hours after sunrise, are usually the most productive for photographers. Many birds are starting their day, and the calmness of the early hours often leads to more predictable behavior.

This is the time when songbirds are most vocal, making it easier to locate them. The gentle light enhances the vibrancy of their plumage, resulting in stunning images. Photographers can take advantage of this time to capture birds in action as they flit between branches or engage in feeding rituals.

On the other hand, late afternoon, especially the final few hours before sunset, provides another excellent opportunity for bird photography. As the day winds down, the lighting becomes warm and golden once again, ideal for capturing the intricate details of feathers and the subtleties of bird behavior.

During this time, birds often return to their roosting spots, making it easier for photographers to observe and photograph them in a relaxed state. The lower angle of the sun also creates long shadows, which can add depth and interest to photographs.

Midday can be challenging for bird photographers due to the harsh overhead sunlight, which can wash out colors and create unflattering shadows. However, this time can still be productive if approached strategically. Birds may seek shelter from the heat, providing opportunities to capture them in shaded areas or near water sources.

Additionally, some species, particularly those in wetlands or coastal areas, may be more active during these hours, allowing for unique photographic opportunities that differ from the early morning and late afternoon routines.

In conclusion, understanding the best times of day for bird photography can significantly influence the quality and success of your images. By planning your shoots around the active periods of birds—early morning and late afternoon—you can take advantage of the optimal lighting conditions and behaviors of the birds.

While midday poses its own challenges, it can also offer unique opportunities if approached with creativity and strategy. Mastering the timing of your photography outings can ultimately lead to more dynamic and compelling images of our avian friends.

Understanding Golden Hour and Blue Hour

Golden Hour and Blue Hour are two critical periods in the daily cycle that every bird photographer should understand and utilize to enhance their images.

Golden Hour occurs shortly after sunrise and just before sunset, characterized by a warm, soft light that bathes the landscape and subjects in a golden hue. This time of day is particularly favorable for bird photography, as the gentle light reduces harsh shadows and highlights, allowing for more even exposure. Birds can often be found more actively foraging or displaying during these times, providing excellent opportunities for capturing dynamic behavior.

Conversely, Blue Hour takes place during the twilight phase, just before sunrise and just after sunset. This period is defined by a cooler, bluish light that can create a serene and ethereal atmosphere in photographs. While the light is dimmer than during Golden Hour, it offers unique opportunities for capturing silhouettes and moody compositions. Birds can be seen flying against the colorful skies, and the overall ambiance can evoke a sense of tranquility, making it an excellent time for artistic interpretations of avian life.

Both Golden Hour and Blue Hour present unique challenges and rewards for photographers. During Golden Hour, the warmth of the light can enhance the colors of a bird's plumage, making it appear more vibrant.

However, the changing light conditions require photographers to adjust their camera settings frequently to avoid overexposure or underexposure.

On the other hand, Blue Hour demands a steady hand or the use of a tripod, as the lower light levels necessitate longer exposure times. Understanding how to manage these conditions, including adjusting ISO and aperture settings, is key to successfully capturing stunning images during these magical hours.

Planning is crucial to make the most of Golden Hour and Blue Hour. Photographers should familiarize themselves with local sunrise and sunset times, as well as weather conditions that may affect light quality. Tools such as smartphone applications can help predict the timing and intensity of these special lighting conditions. Additionally, scouting locations in advance can lead to discovering optimal vantage points to capture birds in their natural habitats against the backdrop of these beautiful times of day.

In conclusion, mastering the art of bird photography during Golden Hour and Blue Hour can significantly elevate the quality of your images. By understanding the characteristics of light during these periods and effectively adapting your techniques, you can create stunning photographs that capture the beauty and essence of avian life. Embrace the challenge of these unique lighting conditions, and let them inspire your creativity as you embark on your journey to master digital bird photography.

Managing Harsh Sunlight and Shadows

Managing harsh sunlight and shadows is crucial for achieving stunning bird photographs. The quality of light in your images can dramatically affect their mood, clarity, and overall impact. When photographing birds, especially in bright sunlight, the light can create harsh contrasts that may obscure details in the feathers and diminish the natural beauty of your subjects. Understanding how to manage these lighting conditions will help you capture the vibrant colors and intricate patterns of birds while minimizing the distractions caused by shadows and glare.

One effective technique for dealing with harsh sunlight is to adjust your shooting schedule. Early mornings and late afternoons, known as the golden hours, provide softer, more diffused light that enhances the colors of birds without the harsh glare that midday sun can produce.

During these times, the angle of the sun is lower, resulting in more flattering light that highlights your subject beautifully. Planning your photography outings around these periods can lead to more visually appealing images.

When shooting in bright sunlight, using reflectors can also help manage shadows and improve lighting conditions. A simple reflector can bounce light onto the bird, filling in shadows and providing a more even exposure. Reflectors come in various materials, including collapsible fabric options that are lightweight and easy to transport.

Positioning the reflector at an angle that catches the sunlight and redirects it towards your subject can significantly enhance your photographs, making colors pop and details more pronounced.

In addition to using reflectors, consider the position of the sun in relation to your subject. Position yourself so that the sun is behind you, illuminating the bird directly. However, this isn't always possible, especially when dealing with skittish species. In such cases, using a lens hood can help reduce lens flare and improve contrast in your images. A lens hood prevents stray light from hitting the lens directly, allowing for clearer, more vibrant photographs even in challenging lighting conditions.

Finally, post-processing can also play a significant role in managing harsh sunlight and shadows. Digital editing software allows you to adjust exposure, contrast, and shadows after the fact, enabling you to salvage images that may have been compromised by extreme lighting conditions. Learning how to effectively use these tools can elevate your photography, allowing you to achieve the desired look even if the original capture wasn't perfect.

By combining these techniques—strategic shooting times, the use of reflectors, proper positioning, and post-processing—you can master the art of capturing birds in all lighting conditions, ensuring your photos are both striking and memorable.

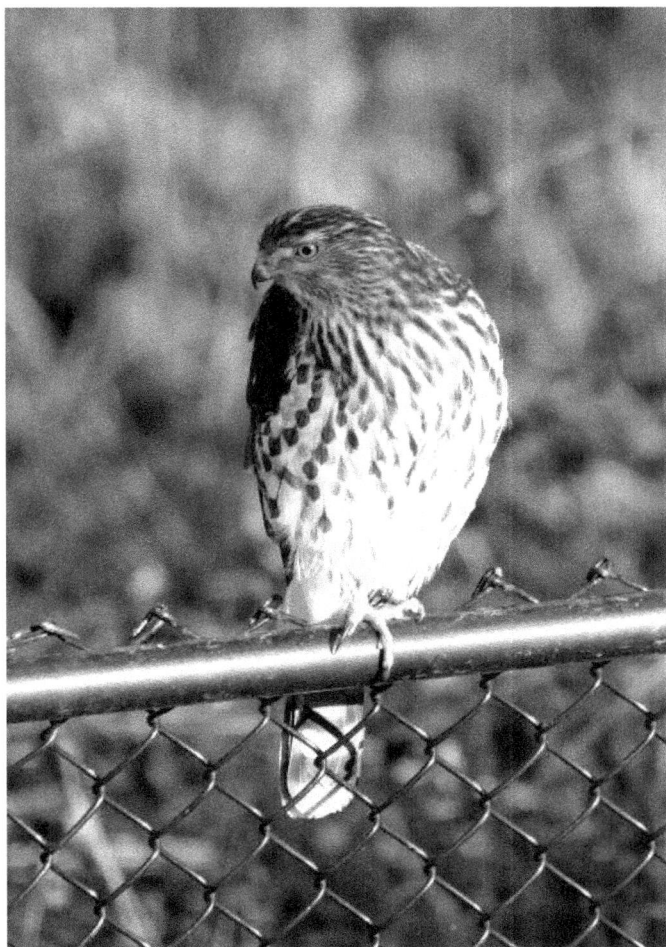

Chapter 7

Field Techniques for Bird Photography

Scouting Locations for Bird Activity

Scouting locations for bird activity is a crucial step in mastering digital bird photography. The right location can significantly enhance your chances of capturing stunning images of your avian subjects. Begin by identifying potential habitats where birds are likely to thrive. These can range from wetlands, forests, and fields to urban parks and gardens. Each environment attracts different species, so understanding the specific needs and behaviors of birds will help you choose the best locations for your photographic endeavors.

Timing is another essential factor in scouting locations. Birds are often most active during the early morning and late afternoon, known as the golden hours of birding. During these times, the lighting is optimal for photography, and the chances of observing various species increase.

Plan your scouting trips to coincide with these peak activity periods. Additionally, consider seasonal changes, as different species migrate or become more prominent in certain habitats throughout the year.

Once you have identified potential locations and timed your visits accordingly, take the time to explore the area thoroughly. Walk quietly and observe the landscape, looking for signs of bird activity such as nests, feeding areas, or flocks in flight. Pay attention to the vegetation and topography, as these elements can influence where and how birds are likely to interact with their environment.

Recording your observations in a notebook or through digital means can help you remember specific spots that yield good results.

Utilizing technology can also enhance your scouting efforts. Mobile apps and websites dedicated to birdwatching can provide insights into recent sightings and popular locations in your area. These tools can help you connect with other bird enthusiasts who may share valuable information about active sites. Additionally, utilizing GPS features can assist you in mapping out your scouting routes and marking promising locations for future visits.

Lastly, patience and persistence are key to successful bird photography. Scouting locations is not just about finding the right spot; it's also about developing a connection with the environment and its inhabitants.

Spend time observing and getting to know the rhythms of the birds in your chosen locations. This understanding will enable you to anticipate their movements and behaviors, ultimately leading to more successful and rewarding photography sessions.

Patience and Stealth in the Field

Patience and stealth are two critical elements in the pursuit of exceptional bird photography. Unlike other subjects that may pose for the camera, birds are often skittish and quick to flee at the slightest hint of disturbance. This makes the photographer's ability to remain patient and undetected essential for capturing stunning images. Understanding the behavior of your avian subjects can significantly enhance your opportunities to photograph them in their natural habitat.

By observing their routines, feeding patterns, and preferred perches, you can position yourself effectively and wait for the perfect moment to click the shutter.

To develop patience in the field, it is vital to adopt a mindset that revels in the experience rather than solely focusing on the end result. Birdwatching can be as rewarding as photography itself, allowing you to appreciate the beauty and intricacies of nature. Spend time in areas where birds are known to frequent, and immerse yourself in the environment.

The more time you dedicate to observing, the more familiar you will become with the habits of your feathered subjects. This familiarity can lead to better opportunities for capturing dynamic shots, as you will be able to anticipate their movements and behaviors.

Stealth is equally important when photographing birds. Moving quietly and minimizing your presence can make a substantial difference in how birds react to you. Wearing neutral-colored clothing that blends into the environment can help you remain inconspicuous. Additionally, consider using natural cover, such as trees or bushes, to conceal your presence.

When setting up your camera, take your time to avoid sudden movements that might startle nearby birds. This deliberate approach can help you get closer to your subjects without alarming them, resulting in more intimate and detailed photographs.

Using the right equipment can also aid in your quest for stealth. A camera with a long lens allows you to shoot from a distance without intruding on the bird's space.

Fast autofocus systems can help you capture quick movements, while silent shutter modes can eliminate noise that might scare birds away. Moreover, carrying lightweight gear will enable you to move more freely and remain agile in the field. By carefully selecting your equipment, you can enhance your ability to remain hidden and ready for those fleeting moments that characterize bird behavior.

Finally, remember that every outing in the field contributes to your skill development as a bird photographer. Patience and stealth are not just techniques but also mindsets that evolve over time. Embrace the process of learning and growing with each experience. The more you practice these principles, the more successful you will become at capturing the beauty of birds in their natural settings. Consistent practice will not only improve your photographic skills but also deepen your connection to the natural world, making every photograph a testament to your dedication and love for bird photography.

Ethical Bird Photography Practices

Ethical bird photography practices are essential for both the welfare of birds and the integrity of the photography community. As photographers, it is our responsibility to ensure that our passion does not negatively impact the subjects we aim to capture. This begins with understanding the habitats of various bird species and the potential disturbances our presence may cause.

Respecting nesting areas and seasonal breeding cycles is crucial. By avoiding sensitive locations during critical times, photographers can help preserve natural behaviors and contribute to the conservation of bird populations.

Using appropriate equipment and techniques is also vital in maintaining ethical standards in bird photography. Telephoto lenses allow you to capture stunning images from a distance, minimizing the need to approach birds closely.

This distance helps prevent stress and disruption to their natural activities. Additionally, employing silent shutter modes and natural light can enhance photo quality while allowing birds to behave more naturally. Understanding the limits of one's equipment and the bird's comfort zone is key to fostering an environment where both the photographer and the subject can coexist harmoniously.

Educating oneself about local wildlife laws and regulations is another fundamental aspect of ethical bird photography. Different regions have specific guidelines designed to protect wildlife and their habitats. Familiarizing oneself with these laws not only helps in avoiding legal issues but also promotes responsible photography practices. Engaging with local wildlife organizations can provide valuable insights into the best practices for photographing birds in particular areas, ensuring that photographers contribute positively to conservation efforts.

Sharing knowledge and promoting ethical practices within the photography community is essential for fostering a culture of responsibility. Photographers can lead by example, showcasing their commitment to ethical practices through their work and interactions with others.

Workshops, online forums, and social media platforms can serve as excellent venues for discussing ethical considerations and sharing experiences. By encouraging dialogue about the importance of respecting wildlife, photographers can inspire others to adopt similar standards, creating a collective impact on the community.

Ultimately, ethical bird photography practices not only enhance the quality of photographs but also contribute to the overall well-being of bird populations and their ecosystems.

By prioritizing the welfare of our subjects and being mindful of our impact, we can capture breathtaking images while ensuring that our actions support conservation and respect for wildlife. Committing to these practices enriches the experience of bird photography, allowing photographers to take pride in their work and its positive influence on the natural world.

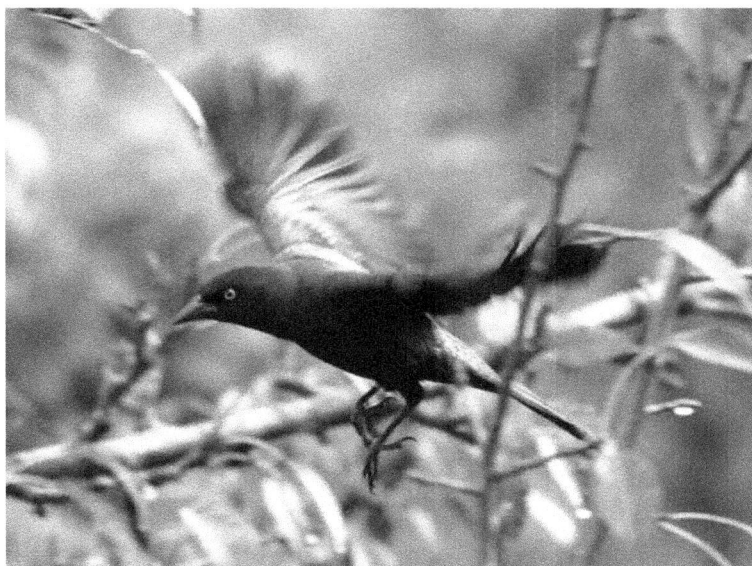

Chapter 8

Post-Processing Your Images

Introduction to Editing Software

Editing software plays a crucial role in the digital photography process, especially for photographers focused on capturing the beauty and intricacies of birds in their natural habitat. With the advent of digital cameras, photographers have more control over their images than ever before.

However, the raw images often require refinement to enhance the visual appeal and to bring out the subtle details that can be lost in the initial capture. Understanding the different types of editing software available is essential for mastering digital bird photography.

There are various editing software options, ranging from basic programs to advanced tools that cater to professional photographers. Programs like Adobe Lightroom and Photoshop are widely recognized in the industry for their powerful features and user-friendly interfaces. Lightroom excels in organizing and processing large batches of images, making it ideal for photographers who shoot numerous photos in a single outing.

On the other hand, Photoshop provides comprehensive editing capabilities, allowing for detailed retouching, layer management, and advanced manipulation techniques that can significantly enhance bird images.

Many photographers may also consider free or lower-cost alternatives, such as GIMP or Paint.NET. These programs, while not as feature-rich as their premium counterparts, offer a solid foundation for beginners looking to improve their editing skills with a less cost.

These options can effectively support basic editing tasks such as cropping, adjusting exposure, and applying filters. As photographers become more comfortable with the editing process, they may find that upgrading to more sophisticated software is beneficial for achieving their artistic vision.

An essential aspect of using editing software is understanding the workflow that best suits individual needs. This includes knowing when to edit images, which adjustments to prioritize, and how to maintain a consistent style throughout a portfolio. For bird photographers, this often means focusing on color correction to capture the vibrant hues of plumage, sharpening details to enhance feather textures, and using cropping techniques to draw attention to the subject. A well-structured workflow can not only streamline the editing process but also elevate the overall quality of the final images.

Ultimately, mastering editing software is a vital skill for anyone passionate about digital bird photography. The ability to refine and enhance images after a shoot allows photographers to convey their artistic vision more effectively and share their work with a broader audience.

By investing time in learning these tools and developing a personal editing style, photographers can transform their raw captures into captivating images that truly reflect the beauty of the avian world.

Basic Editing Techniques for Bird Photos

Basic editing techniques are essential for enhancing bird photographs and bringing out the best in your images. The primary goal of editing is to improve the overall quality of the photograph while maintaining its authenticity.

One of the most fundamental techniques is cropping, which allows photographers to remove distracting elements from the frame and focus the viewer's attention on the bird. Proper cropping can also help improve the composition by adhering to the rule of thirds or other compositional guidelines, ensuring that the bird is positioned in a way that draws the viewer's eye.

Adjusting exposure is another crucial editing technique. Many bird photographs can suffer from overexposure or underexposure due to varying lighting conditions. Using editing software, you can adjust the brightness and contrast to bring out the details in the feathers and surroundings. Increasing contrast can help separate the bird from the background, making it pop and giving the image a more dynamic feel. It's important to be subtle with these adjustments, as overdoing it can lead to unnatural-looking images.

Color correction is vital for achieving accurate and vibrant hues in bird photography. Birds often have intricate color patterns that can be lost in poor lighting or camera settings. By using editing tools to adjust the white balance, you can ensure that the colors are true to life. Saturation adjustments can further enhance the vibrancy of the colors without making them look artificial. It's advisable to compare your edited images to reference photos of the same species to ensure that the colors remain realistic.

Sharpening the image is a technique that can significantly enhance the details in a bird's plumage and features. This process involves increasing the contrast between adjacent pixels to create the illusion of sharper details. However, it's essential to use sharpening selectively, as over-sharpening can result in artifacts that detract from the image's quality. Many editing programs offer localized sharpening tools, allowing you to enhance the bird's features without affecting the entire image.

Finally, noise reduction is an important technique, especially for bird photographers who often shoot in low-light conditions. High ISO settings can introduce unwanted noise, which can distract from the beauty of the bird. Using noise reduction tools in your editing software can help smooth out these imperfections while preserving essential details. Balancing noise reduction with sharpness is crucial; too much noise reduction can make the image look soft or blurry. Mastering these basic editing techniques will enhance your bird photographs, allowing your passion for bird photography to shine through in every image.

Advanced Editing Tips and Tricks

Advanced editing techniques can significantly enhance your digital bird photography, allowing you to showcase the beauty and intricacies of your subjects. One of the first steps in advanced editing is understanding the importance of raw image files.

Shooting in raw format preserves the most data from your camera's sensor, providing greater flexibility in post-processing. This additional data allows for superior adjustments in exposure, white balance, and color without degrading image quality. Familiarizing yourself with the raw editing capabilities of software like Adobe Lightroom or Capture One can transform your workflow and final results.

Color correction is another essential aspect of advanced editing. Birds often display vibrant and varied colors that can sometimes appear flat or misrepresented in photographs. Utilizing tools such as the HSL (Hue, Saturation, and Luminance) sliders allows you to fine-tune individual colors, bringing out the richness and vibrancy of your subject. Additionally, employing selective color adjustments can help in enhancing the colors of the bird while maintaining the natural look of the background. Mastering these techniques can elevate your images, making them more visually striking.

Cropping and composition adjustments also play a vital role in advanced editing. While composition should ideally be considered during the shooting process, post-capture editing provides an opportunity to refine framing. Utilizing the rule of thirds or leading lines can guide the viewer's eye and create a more balanced image.

However, it is crucial to be mindful of the crop factor, as excessive cropping can lead to a loss of detail. Maintaining the integrity of the original image while enhancing the composition is a skill that can be developed with practice.

Noise reduction is often necessary, especially when shooting in low light conditions or at higher ISO settings. Advanced editing software provides specific noise reduction tools that can help preserve detail while minimizing graininess.

It is essential to strike a balance, as over-applying noise reduction can result in a loss of fine details, which is particularly important in bird photography where textures like feathers are critical. Learning how to apply noise reduction selectively can help maintain clarity in your images.

Finally, consider the importance of sharpening your images in post-processing. While it may seem counterintuitive, sharpening should be done with care to enhance the details without introducing artifacts. Use tools that allow you to apply sharpening selectively, focusing on the bird itself while keeping the background soft. This technique draws attention to your subject and enhances the overall impact of the photograph. By mastering these advanced editing tips and tricks, you can significantly improve your digital bird photography, creating images that truly reflect the beauty of your avian subjects.

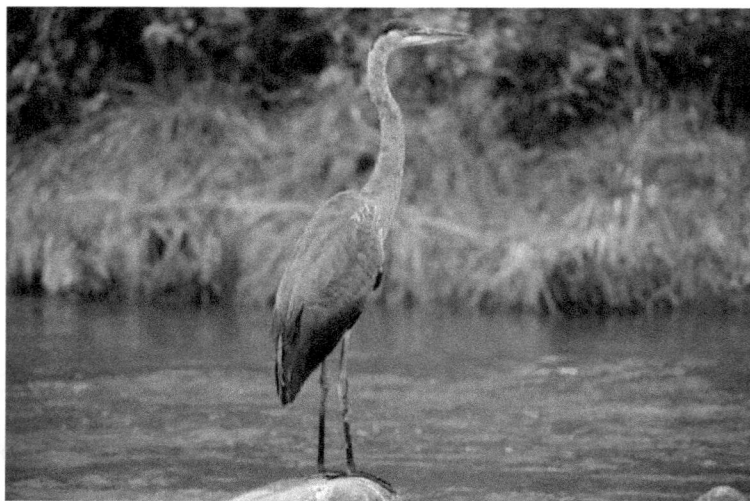

Chapter 9

Sharing and Showcasing Your Work

Creating an Online Portfolio

Creating an online portfolio is an essential step for anyone looking to showcase their passion for digital bird photography. An online portfolio serves as a visual resume, allowing photographers to present their best work while providing a platform for potential clients, collaborators, or enthusiasts to view their skills. It is crucial to choose a user-friendly platform that allows for easy navigation, such as WordPress, Squarespace, or even dedicated photography sites like SmugMug or 500px. Selecting the right platform sets the foundation for a visually appealing and professional presentation.

When curating your portfolio, it is important to focus on quality over quantity. Aim to showcase a selection of your best photographs that highlight your unique style and expertise in bird photography. A well-thought-out collection might include images from different seasons, various bird species, and diverse environments. Consider grouping your images thematically or by location to create a cohesive narrative. This approach not only captivates viewers but also demonstrates your versatility and understanding of the subject matter.

In addition to the photographs themselves, providing context can significantly enhance your portfolio. Adding captions or brief descriptions for each image can help viewers appreciate the story behind the shot, the techniques used, and the challenges faced during the capture. Including information about the camera settings, location, and the behavior of the birds can further engage your audience.

This level of detail showcases your expertise and passion, making your portfolio not just a gallery of images, but a rich resource for those interested in bird photography.

An essential aspect of an online portfolio is the inclusion of an "About Me" section. This is your opportunity to connect with your audience on a personal level. Share your journey into bird photography, your inspirations, and what drives your passion for capturing these beautiful creatures.

Including a professional photograph of yourself can also help to humanize your portfolio and establish a connection with viewers. This personal touch can make your work more relatable and memorable, encouraging visitors to return to your portfolio in the future.

Finally, do not underestimate the importance of promoting your online portfolio. Utilize social media platforms, photography forums, and personal networks to share your work with a larger audience.

Engaging with other photographers and participating in online communities can also help you gain visibility and receive constructive feedback. Regularly updating your portfolio with new work and maintaining an active online presence will keep your audience engaged and interested in your photography journey.

By effectively creating and promoting your online portfolio, you can build a strong foundation for your career as a digital bird photographer.

Social Media Strategies for Photographers

Social media has become an essential tool for photographers, especially those specializing in niche areas like bird photography. It provides an accessible platform to showcase your work, connect with fellow enthusiasts, and engage with potential clients.

To effectively utilize social media, photographers should start by choosing the right platforms that align with their target audience. Instagram, with its visual focus, is particularly effective for showcasing stunning bird images.

Facebook groups dedicated to birdwatching and photography can also be valuable for networking and sharing experiences. By selecting the right platforms, photographers can maximize their reach and impact.

Creating a consistent posting schedule is crucial for maintaining engagement. Regularly sharing high-quality images, behind-the-scenes content, and informative captions keeps your audience interested and encourages them to share your work.

Developing a content calendar helps photographers plan their posts around seasonal events or bird migrations, ensuring that their content remains relevant and timely. This strategy not only boosts visibility but also fosters a sense of community among followers who share similar interests in bird photography.

Engagement is key to building a loyal following on social media. Photographers should actively interact with their audience by responding to comments, asking questions, and encouraging discussions. Engaging with other photographers and bird enthusiasts can lead to collaborations, shout-outs, and increased visibility.

Participating in related hashtags and challenges can further expand reach and allow photographers to connect with a broader audience who shares their passion for bird photography.

Utilizing storytelling in social media posts can also enhance engagement. Sharing the stories behind the photographs, such as the challenges faced during a shoot or the unique behaviors of the birds captured, can create a deeper connection with the audience.

Visual storytelling not only showcases technical skills but also invites viewers to appreciate the beauty of bird life and the dedication required to capture it. This approach encourages followers to invest emotionally in your work, which can lead to increased shares and interactions.

Finally, leveraging analytics tools available on social media platforms can provide valuable insights into audience behavior and content performance. Understanding which posts resonate most with followers allows photographers to refine their strategies and focus on what works best.

By analyzing data such as engagement rates, reach, and demographics, photographers can tailor their content to better meet the interests of their audience, ultimately enhancing their online presence and success in the competitive world of digital bird photography.

Entering Competitions and Exhibitions

Entering competitions and exhibitions can be an exciting step for photographers looking to showcase their work and gain recognition in the field of digital bird photography.

Competitions often offer a platform for photographers to display their skills, creativity, and unique perspectives on avian subjects. Participating in these events can lead to valuable feedback from judges and industry professionals, as well as opportunities for networking with fellow photographers who share a similar passion.

Before entering a competition or exhibition, it's essential to research the various events available. Different competitions may have specific themes, categories, or rules that cater to different styles of bird photography. Some might focus on wildlife conservation, while others may emphasize artistic interpretations.

Understanding the guidelines and criteria for each event will help you select competitions that align with your photographic vision and expertise. This knowledge will also aid in preparing your entries to meet the expectations of the judges.

When preparing your submissions, pay close attention to the technical aspects of your photographs. Ensure your images are not only striking in composition but also technically sound, with proper exposure, sharpness, and color accuracy. Editing plays a vital role in digital photography, so take the time to enhance your images while maintaining a natural look that represents the birds authentically.

Additionally, consider the narrative or story behind each photograph, as compelling narratives can resonate with judges and audiences alike, making your work stand out.

Presentation is another crucial element when entering competitions and exhibitions. Many events require specific formats or sizes for submissions, so adhere strictly to these requirements.

When displaying your work physically, consider matting and framing your photographs professionally to enhance their aesthetic appeal. If the competition allows for digital submissions, ensure that your files are of high resolution and optimized for viewing on screens. A well-presented entry can leave a lasting impression on judges and viewers, highlighting your professionalism as a photographer.

Finally, engaging with the community surrounding competitions and exhibitions can provide further insights and opportunities. Attend openings, workshops, and discussions related to these events to learn from experienced photographers and industry experts. Networking can lead to collaborations, mentorships, and new avenues for showcasing your work. Whether you win or not, the experience of entering competitions and exhibitions can significantly contribute to your growth as a bird photographer, pushing you to refine your skills and expand your creative horizons.

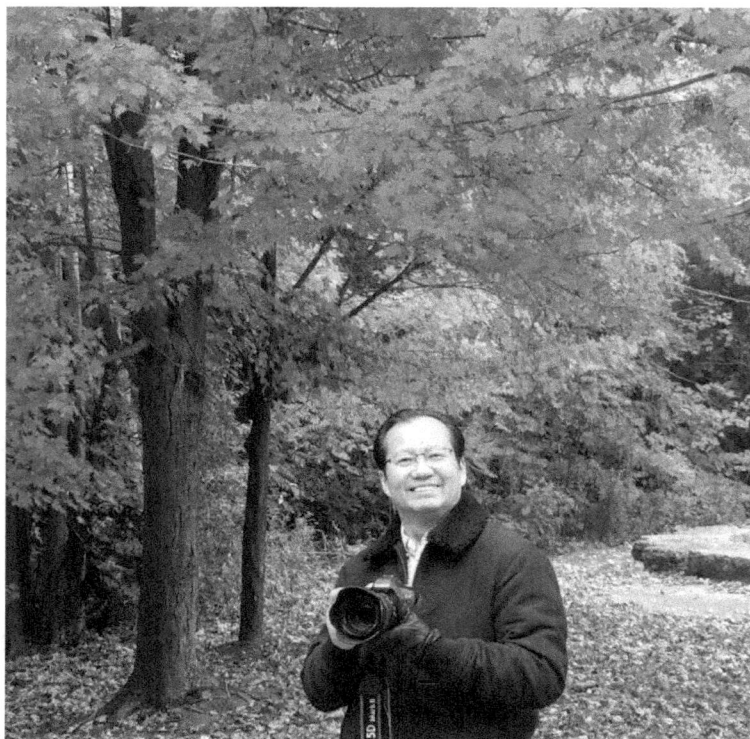

Chapter 10

Continuing Your Bird Photography Journey

Setting Goals for Improvement

Setting goals is a crucial first step in improving your skills in digital bird photography. Without clear objectives, it can be easy to become overwhelmed by the vast array of techniques, equipment, and species to photograph. Start by identifying what specific aspects of bird photography you want to enhance.

This could range from mastering camera settings to improving composition, or even expanding your knowledge of bird behavior to better anticipate their movements. By pinpointing your focus areas, you create a structured path for your growth.

Once you have identified your goals, it is important to make them SMART: Specific, Measurable, Achievable, Relevant, and Time-bound. For instance, instead of stating a vague goal like "I want to take better bird photos," you could set a specific goal such as "I want to capture sharp images of five different species of birds in my local park by the end of the month."

This approach will help you track your progress and make adjustments as needed. Additionally, having a timeline creates a sense of urgency, motivating you to get out and practice regularly.

Another effective strategy for goal-setting is to break larger goals into smaller, manageable tasks. If your larger goal is to master bird photography in various lighting conditions, you can create smaller tasks focusing on each condition.

For example, dedicate one week to shooting in early morning light, and another to shooting during golden hour. This method allows you to focus on one aspect at a time, making it less daunting and more achievable. It also provides you with opportunities to experiment and learn from each specific scenario.

As you work towards your goals, be sure to document your progress. Keeping a photography journal is an excellent way to reflect on what you have learned, note the challenges you face, and celebrate your successes. Take notes on your shooting conditions, camera settings, and any tips or techniques you discover.

This documentation not only reinforces your learning but also provides valuable insights that can inform your future goals. Regularly reviewing your entries will help you identify patterns in your photography and areas that still need improvement.

Finally, consider sharing your goals with a community of fellow bird photographers. Engaging with others who share your passion can provide motivation, support, and accountability. Online forums, social media groups, or local photography clubs can serve as platforms for sharing your experiences and receiving constructive feedback.

By surrounding yourself with like-minded individuals, you can gain new perspectives and inspiration that can further enhance your journey toward mastering digital bird photography.

Joining Photography Communities

Joining photography communities can significantly enhance your journey in mastering digital bird photography. These communities offer a wealth of knowledge, support, and motivation that can transform your skills and approach.

Whether you are a beginner or an experienced photographer, connecting with like-minded individuals can inspire creativity and provide valuable insights into the nuances of capturing avian subjects. Engaging with others who share your passion can foster an environment of learning and growth, making your photography experience more rewarding.

One of the primary benefits of joining photography communities is access to a diverse range of expertise. Members often include seasoned professionals and enthusiastic amateurs who are willing to share their experiences, tips, and techniques.

Many communities host workshops, webinars, and discussions that focus on various aspects of bird photography, from composition and lighting to post-processing techniques.

This collective knowledge can help you refine your skills and discover new methods to enhance your photography. Additionally, receiving feedback on your work from fellow members can provide fresh perspectives that you may not have considered.

Another advantage of being part of a photography community is the opportunity for networking. Building relationships with other photographers can lead to collaborations on projects, such as joint photography outings or exhibitions. These connections can also provide access to exclusive events, such as birdwatching trips or photography contests.

Networking within these communities can open doors to new opportunities, whether it's finding a mentor, gaining exposure for your work, or even discovering potential clients interested in your photography.

Participating in community challenges and competitions can also be a motivating factor. Many photography groups organize monthly themes or contests that encourage members to push their creative boundaries. Engaging in these activities can stimulate your artistic vision and inspire you to experiment with different styles or techniques in your bird photography.

Furthermore, the friendly competition can help you set goals and track your progress, making your photographic journey more structured and goal-oriented.

Lastly, joining a photography community can provide emotional support during challenging times. Photography can often be a solitary pursuit, which may lead to feelings of isolation or self-doubt. Being part of a group that understands your struggles and celebrates your successes can be immensely reassuring.

The camaraderie found in these communities can help you stay motivated and inspired, ensuring that your passion for bird photography continues to flourish. Embracing the community aspect of photography can ultimately enhance not only your skills but also your overall enjoyment of the craft.

Resources for Ongoing Learning and Inspiration

To truly master digital bird photography, ongoing learning and inspiration are essential components. Resources such as books, online courses, and workshops can provide valuable insights into techniques, equipment, and artistic expression. Engaging with these resources not only enhances technical skills but also fosters a deeper understanding of avian behavior, which is crucial for capturing stunning images.

Exploring a variety of formats allows photographers to tailor their learning experiences to their preferences and schedules.

Books remain one of the most reliable resources for photographers at all levels. There are numerous titles that focus specifically on bird photography, offering advice on everything from composition and lighting to understanding bird habits.

Authors often share their personal experiences, which can be both educational and motivating. Additionally, field guides can assist photographers in identifying bird species and understanding their habitats, enriching the overall photographic experience.

Online courses have gained popularity due to their accessibility and variety. Websites dedicated to photography often host classes taught by experienced photographers.

These courses can range from beginner to advanced levels, covering essential topics such as camera settings, lens selection, and post-processing techniques. Participants can also benefit from community forums where they can share their work, ask questions, and receive feedback from peers and instructors. This interactive element helps build a supportive learning environment.

Workshops provide hands-on experience that can significantly enhance skills and confidence. Many professional photographers offer workshops in natural settings, allowing participants to practice their craft while receiving real-time guidance. These immersive experiences are invaluable for learning how to approach birds in their habitats, understand the importance of patience, and develop an eye for capturing fleeting moments. Networking with other photographers during workshops can also lead to lasting connections and opportunities for collaboration.

Lastly, online communities and social media platforms have become vital sources of inspiration and knowledge. Joining photography groups allows enthusiasts to share their work, exchange tips, and discuss challenges. Following professional photographers on platforms like Instagram and YouTube can provide daily doses of inspiration as well as practical advice.

Engaging with these communities can motivate photographers to continue improving their skills and exploring new creative avenues, ensuring a lifelong journey of learning in the realm of digital bird photography.

Author Notes & Acknowledgments

First and foremost, I would like to express my deepest gratitude to the people who inspired and supported me throughout the journey of writing this book. This project would not have been possible without their unwavering belief in me and their invaluable contributions.

To my wife, thank you for your constant encouragement and understanding. Your love and support have been my anchor during the challenging times of researching and writing this book.

I would also like to disclose that this book contains some renewed artificial intelligence-generated content. I really appreciate very recent technological innovation by outstanding scientists and of course our reader's understanding.

Lastly, I want to express my deepest gratitude to the readers of this book.I sincerely hope the strategies and methods outlined within these pages will provide you with the knowledge and tools needed to truly make your life much better. Your commitment to seeking any good solutions and willingness to explore multiple methods is commendable.

Author Bio

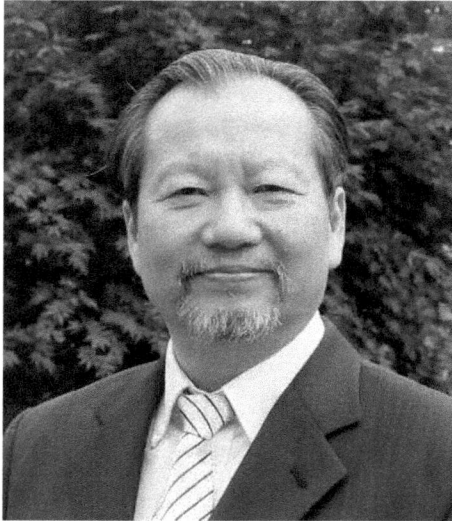

Johnson Wu is an experienced bird photographer with an enthusiastic passion for digital photography. He has gained extensive knowledge from professionals in the field and has accumulated significant experience in capturing stunning bird images. Over the years, Johnson has photographed numerous bird species, producing exceptional images across a wide variety of them.

In addition to his passion for photography, Johnson Wu earned his MD in 1982 and has worked in hospitals in both China and the UK. Upon the recommendation of Sir Aaron Klug, the former president of The Royal Society and Nobel Prize winner in Chemistry, Dr. Wu was honored with a British Royal Society Fellowship. He has published over 100 medical books and currently practices medicine in Canada.

www.ingramcontent.com/pod-product-compliance
Lightning Source LLC
Chambersburg PA
CBHW060239030426

42335CB00014B/1531